MELATONIN

A Beginner's 3-Week Guide on How
to Leverage Melatonin for Anti-Aging,
Sleep Quality, and Brain Health

Tyler Spellmann

mindplusfood

Copyright © 2021 Tyler Spellmann

All rights reserved
No part of this book may be reproduced, or stored in a retrieval system, or transmitted in any form or by any means, electronic, mechanical, photocopying, recording, or otherwise, without express written permission of the publisher.

Printed in the United States of America

CONTENTS

Title Page
Copyright
Disclaimer
Introduction — 1
Sleep 101 — 3
What You Need to Know About Melatonin — 7
Week 1 — 14
Week 2 — 16
Week 3 — 20
Sample Recipes — 22
Conclusion — 34
Reference and Helpful Links — 35

DISCLAIMER

By reading this disclaimer, you are accepting the terms of the disclaimer in full. If you disagree with this disclaimer, please do not read the guide.

All of the content within this guide is provided for informational and educational purposes only, and should not be accepted as independent medical or other professional advice. The author is not a doctor, physician, nurse, mental health provider, or registered nutritionist/dietician. Therefore, using and reading this guide does not establish any form of a physician-patient relationship.

Always consult with a physician or another qualified health provider with any issues or questions you might have regarding any sort of medical condition. Do not ever disregard any qualified professional medical advice or delay seeking that advice because of anything you have read in this guide. The information in this guide is not intended to be any sort of medical advice and should not be used in lieu of any medical advice by a licensed and qualified medical professional.

The information in this guide has been compiled from a variety of known sources. However, the author cannot attest to or guarantee the accuracy of each source and thus should not be held liable for any errors or omissions.

You acknowledge that the publisher of this guide will not be held liable for any loss or damage of any kind incurred as a result of this guide or the reliance on any information provided within this guide. You acknowledge and agree that you assume all risk and responsibility for any action you undertake in response to the information in this guide.

Using this guide does not guarantee any particular result (e.g., weight loss or a cure). By reading this guide, you acknowledge that there are no guarantees to any specific outcome or results you can expect.

All product names, diet plans, or names used in this guide are for identification purposes only and are the property of their respective owners. The use of these names does not imply endorsement. All other trademarks cited herein are the property of their respective owners.

Where applicable, this guide is not intended to be a substitute for the original work of this diet plan and is, at most, a supplement to the original work for this diet plan and never a direct substitute. This guide is a personal expression of the facts of that diet plan.

Where applicable, persons shown in the cover images are stock photography models and the publisher has obtained the rights to use the images through license agreements with third-party stock image companies.

INTRODUCTION

Gone are the days when people stop working at exactly 5 pm and sleep at 8 pm to complete 8 to 10 hours worth of sleep. The hustle and bustle of life penetrated our lives so much that most of us have developed a comfort zone in moving and working most of our time.

Pausing from our usual daily activities does not come naturally anymore. It takes deliberate practice to sit down and meditate for even just a few minutes of our time. However, did you know that sleep is just as important as diet and exercise?

Our mind and body are active 24/7, so a decrease in energy consumption for 8 hours a day is the least that we can do to recover from the daily stress of life.

As much as everyone would want to go to bed on time, it does not always come easy. For some, falling asleep is as fast as counting 1, 2, 3. Whereas for others, it takes effort and practice. This could be because of different factors such as diet before bedtime, sleeping habits, and genetic predispositions.

Some may have a shorter biological clock while others may have it longer than 24 hours a day.

Some may also have lower levels of melatonin making it difficult for them to achieve a good quality of sleep on a nightly basis.

If you are one of those who toss and turn in bed a lot and find it a challenge to get some good sleep, continue reading this guide to learn how melatonin might be the solution to your problem.

In this guide, you will:
- Understand the importance of sleep.
- Learn what melatonin is and why it is important.
- Check if you are one of those who need a daily dose of melatonin.
- Discover the other health benefits of melatonin.
- Familiarize yourself with melatonin-containing foods.

SLEEP 101

Why do we need to sleep? To appreciate and understand why we need melatonin, let us first dive into the importance of sleep.

If computers overheat and conk out when overused, what more for the human body that has to stay functional and alive for at least 70 years? Just like computers, our bodies need a reset to be able to:

• Synthesize macromolecules
• Repair vesicles, substances, and membranes of our cells needed in maintaining balance in our body
• Reorganize neural networks and consolidate memory
• Restore immune function

Sleep is an "active state of unconsciousness"; wherein, our body actively shuts down as a response to internal and external stimuli. However, up to this day, sleep remains to be a mystery in a lot of aspects.

Scientists have time and time again tried to measure sleep and explain fully why we need it. However, all we have at the moment are theories that are bound to be proven false or true.

Energy Conservation Theory
Sleep is important because we need to conserve energy when we are least expected to hunt for food.

Taking an 8-hour break from our busy life is needed to reduce our body's demand for energy. An 8-hour sleep can slow down the process of generating energy by 15-30%, in turn, decreasing the total energy expenditure of our body by 5-15%.

Restorative Theory
While our body is resting, our body restores what we have used up or lost while we were awake. While we are asleep, the following occur:
- muscle growth
- tissue repair
- protein synthesis
- growth hormone release

During our waking hours, our cells leave a by-product called "adenosine." This adenosine accumulates as we remain awake. The build-up of this by-product is what makes us feel tired and sleepy at the end of the day.

An intake of caffeine is only able to block the effect of adenosine from making us feel sleepy. This is why we can stay alert only up to a certain period.

Sleep, on the other hand, removes the build-up of adenosine making us stay awake for hours.

Brain Plasticity Theory
Did you ever experience thinking of a problem before going to bed and dreaming about the solution? This theory can be used to explain that mystery.
It revolves around the idea that the brain can reorganize neural

connections and consolidate memory. Thus, the solution to your problem could just be lurking behind your thoughts and memories. All you have to do is sleep.

This is also why infants need to sleep for at least 14 hours to allow their brains to grow anatomically and mature physiologically.

Other Benefits of Sleep

- Mental Health

Scott et al. discussed in their study that sleep and mental health have a bidirectional relationship.

Meaning, chronic lack of sleep can lead to disturbances in mental health and vice versa. One example is the relationship between insomnia and depression as measured in the same study. Patients with insomnia developed depression, and those with depression suffered from insomnia.

On the other side of the spectrum, complete sleep can lead to mental gains. Sleep can improve emotional well-being by stimulating the following areas:
- Amygdala
- Striatum
- Hippocampus
- Insula
- Medial prefrontal complex

- Weight Management

Two known hormones signal hunger and fullness. These are ghrelin for hunger and leptin for fullness.

Some reports say that those who sleep less than 7.7 hours a night have a higher BMI average, higher ghrelin levels, and lower leptin levels.

The explanation for this is that when you are awake, ghrelin sends a message to the hypothalamic-pituitary axis of the brain that the body is hungry and needs energy for the body to remain functional.

On the contrary, while asleep, leptin levels increase signaling the body that there is no need to resupply energy.

WHAT YOU NEED TO KNOW ABOUT MELATONIN

What is melatonin and how is it connected to circadian rhythms?

Some are blessed and can initiate and maintain sleep effortlessly for 8 hours a night. Unfortunately, some are on the opposite side of the spectrum and cannot seem to fall asleep no matter how many sheep they count at night.

Why is this so?

We are more primal than we think we are—our bodies are governed by instincts and reflexes. One of these is the circadian rhythm, or the sleep-wake cycle, just like all the other animals in the kingdom.

It is a 24-hour internal clock that influences our level of alertness and behavior telling us when to sleep, wake up, and eat.

How does this work?

Our eyes have two kinds of photoreceptors in our retina (back wall of the eyeballs) called the rods and cones.

These two photoreceptors work in tandem to receive "light" in the daytime and "darkness" in the nighttime. The received information is transmitted to the master clock in the brain called the suprachiasmatic nucleus (SCN) which is found in the hypothalamus.

From the information received, the master clock creates a series of instructions for the body. One of which is the release or suppression of melatonin.

At night, when less light enters the eyes, the brain signals the master clock or SCN, which instructs the pineal gland to produce melatonin and release it into the bloodstream. This production of melatonin results in sleepiness and drowsiness.

Who needs melatonin?

As mentioned earlier, melatonin is a sleep hormone released by the master clock or SCN in response to darkness. Although melatonin is naturally produced in the pineal gland, there are those who need exogenous melatonin as a supplement.

Elderly
Researchers speculate that the SCN loses control over circadian rhythms in advancing age. This is seen in some studies that show that melatonin production peaks at the age of 8 to 10 and gradually declines during puberty. By the age of 40 to 45, the production of melatonin declines faster. By the age of 70, only ~10% of melatonin levels remain.

This is why 50% to 70% of the elderly complain of difficulty falling and staying asleep, and waking up too early in the morning.

Sleep Disorders

Human beings vary in melatonin levels making it more difficult for others to fall asleep.

One of the most common is Delayed Sleep-Wake Phase Disorder. Those with this disorder have difficulty sleeping before 2 am to 6 am and usually wake up between 10 am to 1 pm.

More research is needed to explain and pinpoint the origin of sleep disorders. Although causality is still unclear, evidence shows that there is a strong correlation between sleep disorders and mental health. Most of those who suffer from DSWPD are teenagers and have underlying mental health issues.

Travelers and Shift Workers
Crossing time zones and working at night adjust the sleep-wake cycle. This adjustment makes it a challenge for some to go back to their normal cycle affecting their alertness, mood, and productivity.

Individuals Experiencing Pre-surgery Anxiety
For those who are about to undergo a surgical procedure, taking melatonin before the operation can decrease anxiety. Studies even show that the results are at par with Midazolam, which is a prescription anxiolytic drug.

What are the benefits?

Thermoregulation
One of the physiological functions that occur while we are asleep is a change in body temperature. The body deliberately decreases our temperature to conserve energy. Aside from this, a low body temperature keeps you asleep more comfortably at night.

Melatonin is one of the important contributors that signals the master clock to regulate body temperature at bedtime. One study found that the lowest drop in body temperature was seen within 2 hours before bedtime.

Comorbidities

Hypertension
You might be wondering why there are anti-hypertensive drugs that keep you awake at night (e.g. beta-blockers). This is because they reduce the production of melatonin in your pineal gland.

Studies say that a daily dose of 2mg to 3mg prolonged-release of melatonin can remarkably improve nighttime blood pressure and help those on antihypertensives fall asleep faster and stay asleep longer at night.

Diabetes Mellitus
In general, increasing melatonin intake can decrease inflammatory biomarkers in metabolic syndrome. How? No one knows for sure yet. There is still a lot of confusion in this area.

However, despite the lack of research, some theories suggest that the melatonin receptor, MTNR1B, plays a role in blood glucose levels linking Type 2 Diabetes Mellitus and decreased levels of melatonin.

This is supported by some data that show that diabetics suffering from nerve weakness and pains also have decreased levels of melatonin contributing to their chronic insomnia.

Supplementing with melatonin, they did not only address insomnia but also improved blood sugar levels.

Sexual Development and Reproductive Cycle
Melatonin is an important precursor in sexual maturation and normal reproductive functions in puberty and pregnancy.

Evidence shows that melatonin supplementation can even decrease oxidative damage in ovarian follicles, which boosts fertility and increases the chances of getting pregnant.

Antioxidant and Anti-Inflammatory
There are a lot of speculations that say that melatonin has anti-aging effects. Perhaps, these assumptions stem from its antioxidant and anti-inflammatory properties.

Melatonin is able to scavenge reactive oxygen and nitrogen species that are known to damage cells. Multiple studies have shown that melatonin can fight off oxidative stress and resist inflammation and cell death.

Cancer
Melatonin can be used as an additional treatment for cancers such as breast, prostate, gastric, and colorectal. It can strengthen the effects of chemotherapy and radiotherapy, inhibit tumor growth, and lessen adverse effects from their ongoing treatment. By also improving the quality of sleep of cancer patients, quality of life follows.

What are the risks?

Melatonin is one of the safest supplements out on the market with only mild adverse effects.

These are:
- Headache
- Dizziness
- Nausea
- Sleepiness

If you are thinking of having a daily dose of melatonin, you have little to worry about.

Are there special precautions?

This section applies to melatonin supplementation only. Even if there are minimal reported side effects, it does not mean that we can take melatonin supplements without being careful. Short-term intake of melatonin supplementation has been reported to be generally safe, but long-term use is still questionable.

It might be tempting to pop in another dose whenever you can't sleep at night. However, if low-dose melatonin does not work for you, see your doctor for alternatives and other techniques instead of overdosing.

Remember that melatonin is a hormone. Meaning, it sends messages throughout your system to maintain balance. If you have less or more of it, it can cause harmful effects.

Here are a few things you might want to consider before taking a daily dose:

Drug Interactions
If you are taking maintenance medicines, ask your primary physician first if you can take melatonin. It might decrease or increase the effects of your current medications.

Especially if you are taking the following:
- Blood-thinners
- Anticonvulsants
- Immunosuppressants
- Diabetes Drugs
- Antihypertensives
- Contraceptive pills

Allergy
Be aware of your allergens and check if you are allergic to melatonin. There are some reports of hypersensitivity reactions to melatonin.

Elderly with Dementia

Compared to the younger population, there is a possibility that melatonin can linger in the elderly's system making them groggy in the daytime. This is especially observed in patients who suffer from dementia. This is why the American Academy of Sleep Medicine does not recommend melatonin for patients with dementia.

Trusted Brand
Look for a trusted brand that discloses the ingredients of their products because some include serotonin in their supplements, which can cause harmful effects.

WEEK 1

Checklist
Before anything, we have to start with the basics. This includes developing your sleep hygiene and healthy daily practices and removing habits that negatively affect your sleep-wake cycle.

Below is a checklist that you can start practicing to be able to develop a more sustainable sleeping habit:

• Expose yourself to sunlight during the day so that your brain knows that it is daytime. By doing this every day, your body clock will eventually synchronize with daylight and nighttime darkness.

• Exercising during the day is preferable to a nighttime workout. Using up your energy in the daytime will help you get tired and sleepy at night. However, if unavoidable, only do light to moderate exercises at least an hour before bedtime to give your heart rate enough time to settle and your core body temperature to cool down.

• Budget your naps. Oversleeping in the daytime can make it harder for you to fall asleep at night. Keep your naps less than 30 minutes and make sure not to have them in the late afternoon.

• Avoid taking caffeine in the late afternoon because it can stay in your system longer than you think, making it harder for you to initiate sleep.

• Dim your lights an hour before bedtime to cue your brain that it is time for winding down.

• Practice a routine before going to bed like meditating, listening to soft music, and reading a book. If this is done consistently, the brain will pick up the cue and will follow suit.

• Keep all your devices an hour before bedtime because the blue light being emitted by your gadget can falsely signal the brain that it's still daytime.

• Deliberately make your sleeping environment comfortable. This can be done by keeping your pillows as soft as you want them to be, having clean linens, adjusting your room temperature, or spraying some lavender to induce relaxation.

Remember not to let go of your healthy habits as you progress in your practice. Your habits must remain intact so that you do not relapse into your old ways and desynchronize your sleep-wake cycle.

WEEK 2

Shopping List
Now that you have started to train your brain and body, it is time to add some boost.

There are four vitamins that promote sleep: Tryptophan, Magnesium, Calcium, and Vitamin B6.

You can increase the intake of foods that contain any of these four at a particular time to promote sleepiness.

Tryptophan
A known amino acid that is converted into serotonin and then to melatonin. It is found in:
- Dairy products
- Fruits
- Grains
- Legumes
- Nuts and seeds
- Poultry
- Seafood
- Vegetables

Calcium
Calcium is needed to produce melatonin. By increasing calcium stores, you can also increase melatonin secretion. This is found in:

- Broccoli
- Cheeses
- Dark leafy greens
- Enriched bread and grains
- Fortified cereals
- Fortified orange juice
- Green snap peas
- Low-fat milk
- Okra
- Sardines
- Soybeans
- Yogurt

Vitamin B6 or Pyridoxal 5'-Phosphate
Did you know that those with depression and other mood disorders have low vitamin B6? This is because vitamin B6 helps tryptophan to convert into serotonin and melatonin.

You can find this in:
- Avocado
- Bananas
- Dried Prunes
- Fish: tuna, salmon, and halibut
- Flaxseed
- Meat
- Pistachio nuts
- Spinach
- Sunflower seeds

Melatonin
If you want a direct boost of your melatonin, here are some food sources that you might want to add to your diet:
- Fruits and vegetables: asparagus, broccoli, corn, cucumber, grapes, olives, pomegranate, tart cherries, tomatoes,
- Grains: barley, rice, rolled oats
- Nuts and seeds: flaxseed, mustard, peanuts, sunflower seeds,

seeds, walnuts

Beverages
If you want to have a hot cup of drink before bed, here are some beverages that can help get a good night's sleep:
- Almond milk
- Chamomile tea
- Passion fruit tea
- Peppermint tea
- Tart cherry juice
- Valerian tea

Avoid Before Bedtime
If there are foods that promote sleepiness, there are also those that you need to avoid before going to bed that can potentially induce wakefulness.

Caffeine
Whenever you drink a cup of coffee or caffeinated tea, it blocks your adenosine from binding to the adenosine receptors in the brain. Without this binding, melatonin production in the pineal gland is hindered. Hence, the effect of staying awake, is thus it would be smarter not to drink coffee late in the afternoon.

It might also be wiser to start limiting your daily coffee intake because drinking more than 3 cups of coffee every day for 20 years can shrink your pineal gland and decrease melatonin production.

Spicy Food
Aside from getting possible indigestion or an upset tummy in bed, a study was able to show that those who consumed tabasco took longer to fall asleep and enter phase 2 of sleep. It was noted that their body temperature was higher than usual which could have influenced their sleep stages.

Alcohol

Although alcohol is a downer and can make you sleepy, it can disrupt your progress into the deeper stages of sleep. This prevents complete restoration of energy making you feel sleepy the following morning.

Some say that drinking alcohol starts a cycle of drinking caffeine during the day and consuming more alcohol at night to induce sleepiness. This cycle is the reason why most alcoholics suffer from insomnia.

Fatty Food
Studies discovered that if you consume more fat at night, you are most likely to wake up more in the middle of your sleep and spend less time in REM (Rapid Eye Movement), which is a stage that is important for memory consolidation, enhancing neural connections, and mind restoration.

Too Much Water
This is pretty much self-explanatory. If you drink a lot of water at night, you will end up heading to the toilet now and then interrupting your sleep. Although water will keep you hydrated while you are asleep, best to time it correctly by taking your last sip an hour or two before bedtime.

WEEK 3

Now that you:
✓ understand the importance of sleep
✓ know what melatonin is and why it is important
✓ have checked if you are one of those who need a daily dose of melatonin
✓ are aware of the other health benefits of melatonin
✓ have familiarized yourself with melatonin-containing foods.

It is time to prepare meals that you can have for dinner to increase melatonin before bedtime.

Sample Schedule

	PM Snack/ Appetizer	Dinner
Monday	Asian Zucchini Salad	Lemon-Baked Salmon Tomato and Basil Soup
Tuesday	Kale Salad with Strawberry & Almonds	Turkey Sandwich
Wednesday	Orange- Walnut Salad	Salmon and Asparagus
Thursday	Salmon Soup	Tomato Clams
Friday	Avocado Fruit Salad with Tangerine Vinaigrette	Baked Salmon

SAMPLE RECIPES

Asian Zucchini Salad

Ingredients:
- 1 medium zucchini, sliced thinly into spirals
- 1/3 cup rice vinegar
- 3/4 cup avocado oil
- 1 cup sunflower seeds, shells removed
- 1 lb. cabbage, shredded
- 1 tsp. stevia drops
- 1 cup almonds, sliced

Instructions:
1. Cut the zucchini spirals into smaller parts. Set aside.
2. Put almonds, sunflower seeds, and cabbage in a large bowl. Combine the ingredients well.
4. Add zucchini to the mixture.
5. In a small bowl, mix vinegar, stevia, and oil using a whisk or fork.
6. Pour the vinegar mixture all over the zucchini mixture. Toss well. Make sure everything is covered with the dressing.
7. Refrigerate for 2 hours before serving.

Lemon-Baked Salmon

Ingredients:
- 2 pcs. lemons, thinly sliced
- 3 lbs. salmon filet
- kosher salt
- black pepper, freshly ground
- 6 tbsp. butter, melted, 6 tbsp.
- 2 tbsp. honey
- 3 cloves garlic, minced
- 1 tsp. thyme leaves, chopped
- 1 tsp. dried oregano
- fresh parsley, chopped, for garnish

Instructions:
1. Preheat the oven to 350°F.
2. Line a rimmed baking sheet with foil. Grease with cooking oil spray.
3. Lay lemon slices on the center of the foil.
4. Season salmon filets on both sides with kosher salt and freshly ground black pepper.
5. Place the filet on top of the lemon slices.
6. Whisk together oregano, thyme, garlic, honey, and butter in a small bowl.
7. Pour the mixture over the salmon filet.
8. Fold the foil up and around the salmon to form a packet.
9. Bake for 25 minutes or until the salmon is cooked through.
10. Switch to broil and continue cooking for 2 more minutes.
11. Garnish with chopped fresh parsley and serve hot.

Tomato and Basil Soup

Ingredients:
- 1 medium-sized onion, chopped
- 1 clove garlic, sliced finely
- 2 tablespoons olive oil
- 3 pcs. vine tomatoes or 8 pcs. cherry tomatoes, chopped
- 400 g can plum tomatoes
- 150 ml water
- 5 leaves of fresh basil or 1 tsp. dried basil
- 1 tsp. salt
- pepper

Instructions:
1. Sauté onion, tomatoes, garlic, and basil in olive oil.
2. Pour in the canned tomatoes. Add salt and pepper.
3. Cover and let it simmer for 30 minutes on low heat.
4. Transfer to a blender or food processor and blend until smooth.
5. Serve and enjoy.

Kale Salad with Strawberry and Almonds

Ingredients:
- 1 bunch of kale
- 1/2 cup sliced strawberries
- 1/4 cup sliced almonds
- 1 lemon pulp juice
- 1/8 tsp. salt
- 1/8 tsp. black pepper
- 1 tbsp. agave
- 2 tbsp. of olive oil

Instructions:
1. Rip kale into small pieces and massage with hands until tender.
2. Put it in a bowl. Add almonds and strawberries.
3. To create a dressing, mix lemon juice with olive oil, salt, pepper, and agave, and then pour it over the salad.
4. Serve immediately.

Turkey Sandwich

Ingredients:
- 3 oz. roasted turkey, sliced
- 2 oz. whole wheat pita bread
- a few pcs. romaine lettuce leaves
- 1 tsp. mustard
- 2 slices tomato
- 1/2 cup grapes, cut in half

Instructions:
1. Cut pita bread in half, fully opening the pocket in the middle.
2. Layer the ingredients inside each pita bread slice.
3. Briefly heat in the microwave oven or on a pan if desired.
4. Serve and enjoy while warm.

Orange-Walnut Salad

Ingredients:
- 2 cups romaine lettuce, chopped coarsely
- 1 cucumber, peeled and deseeded, quartered lengthwise and chopped
- 1 cup arugula
- 2 navel oranges, peeled and chopped
- 1/4 cup red onion, sliced thinly
- 1 tbsp. walnut oil
- 2 tbsp. walnuts, chopped
- 1 tbsp. red wine vinegar
- 2 oz. blue cheese, gluten-free

Instructions:
1. In a salad bowl, carefully place the ingredients into layers.
2. Sprinkle with walnut oil and vinegar and toss.
3. With your hands, crumble blue cheese on top.
4. Serve immediately and enjoy.

Salmon and Asparagus

Ingredients:
- 2 salmon filets
- 14-oz. young potatoes
- 8 asparagus spears, trimmed and halved
- 2 handfuls cherry tomatoes
- 1 handful basil leaves
- 2 tbsp. extra-virgin olive oil
- 1 tbsp. balsamic vinegar

Instructions:
1. Heat oven to 428°F.
2. Arrange potatoes into a baking dish.
3. Drizzle potatoes with extra-virgin olive oil.
4. Roast potatoes until they have turned golden brown.
5. Place asparagus into the baking dish together with the potatoes.
6. Roast in the oven for 15 minutes.
7. Arrange cherry tomatoes and salmon among the vegetables.
8. Drizzle with balsamic vinegar and the remaining olive oil.
9. Roast until the salmon is cooked.
10. Throw in basil leaves before transferring everything to a serving dish.
11. Serve while hot.

Tomato Clams

Ingredients:
- Canola oil cooking spray
- 1 onion, sliced
- 1 tsp. minced garlic, or to taste
- 1/2 tsp salt
- 3 pounds of clams, in shell, thoroughly scrubbed
- 1 tsp red pepper flakes
- 1 cup white wine
- 1/2 lb. whole-grain linguine, cooked according to package directions
- 1/2 cup flat-leaf parsley, chopped
- 4 cups cherry tomatoes, halved

Instructions:
1. Heat a large pot with a lid over low heat.
2. Spray with vegetable oil cooking spray and add the onion, garlic, and salt. Cook for 3 minutes, stirring constantly.
3. Add the clams, red pepper flakes, and wine
4. Cover and simmer until the clams open, approximately 7 minutes. Discard those clams that do not open.
5. Add the pasta, parsley, and tomatoes. Cover and let simmer for an additional 3 minutes. Stir and serve immediately.

Salmon Soup

Ingredients:
- 1-3/4 cup coconut milk
- 2 tsp. dried thyme leaves
- 4 leeks, trimmed and sliced into crescents
- 6 cups seafood stock or chicken broth
- salt, for seasoning
- 3 cloves garlic, minced
- 1 lb. salmon, cut into bite-sized pieces
- 2 tbsp. avocado oil

Instructions:
1. Place avocado oil in a large saucepan or Dutch oven at low-medium heat. Add garlic and leeks.
2. Cook vegetables until slightly softened.
3. Pour in chicken or fish stock. Add in thyme and allow the mixture to simmer for approximately 15 minutes.
4. Season with salt to taste.
5. Add both coconut milk and salmon.
6. Bring the mixture up to a gentle simmer.
7. Cook until the fish is tender and opaque, then serve while hot.

Fruit Salad with Zesty Vinaigrette

Ingredients:
- 3 mangoes, medium-sized, peeled and sliced thinly
- 3 ripe avocados, medium-sized, peeled and thinly sliced
- 1 cup blackberries, fresh
- 1 cup raspberries, fresh
- 1/4 cup mint, fresh and minced
- 1/4 cup almonds, toasted and sliced

For the dressing:
- 1 tsp. tangerine, grated, or orange peel
- 1/2 cup olive oil
- 1/2 tsp. salt
- 1/4 cup juice from a tangerine or an orange
- 1/4 tsp. freshly ground pepper
- 2 tbsp. balsamic vinegar

Instructions:
1. Combine all the fruits on a serving plate.
2. Sprinkle the salad with mint and almonds.
3. Whisk together all the dressing ingredients in a smaller bowl.
4. Drizzle the dressing over the salad.
5. Consume after serving.

Baked Salmon

Ingredients:
- 2 salmon fillets
- 6 cups of fresh spinach
- 2 tsp. coconut oil
- 1/4 tsp. garlic powder
- 1/4 tsp. turmeric
- 3 large cloves of garlic
- lemon juice
- salt
- pepper

Instructions:
1. Preheat the oven to 400°F.
2. Line a baking dish with parchment paper.
3. Marinate salmon fillets in lemon juice, coconut oil, garlic powder, turmeric, salt, and pepper.
4. Let it sit for a few minutes. This may also be done the night before to help the juices and flavor get into the salmon.
5. Once the oven is ready, bake the salmon for 15 minutes.
6. Cook some of the garlic in a pan with coconut oil.
7. Add spinach and cook until ready. Season with salt and pepper to taste.
8. Take salmon out of the oven and put spinach beside it.
9. Serve and enjoy.

CONCLUSION

Thank you again for getting this guide.

If you found this guide helpful, please take the time to share your thoughts and post a review. It'd be greatly appreciated!

Thank you and good luck!

REFERENCE AND HELPFUL LINKS

Alcohol and sleep. (2020, September 4). Sleep Foundation. https://www.sleepfoundation.org/nutrition/alcohol-and-sleep.

Garaulet, M., Qian, J., Florez, J. C., Arendt, J., Saxena, R., & Scheer, F. A. J. L. (2020). Melatonin effects on glucose metabolism: Time to unlock the controversy. Trends in Endocrinology & Metabolism, 31(3), 192–204. https://doi.org/10.1016/j.tem.2019.11.011.

Is it bad to take melatonin every night? Are there risks? (2020, November 6). Healthline. https://www.healthline.com/health/is-it-bad-to-take-melatonin-every-night.

Karasek, M. (2004). Melatonin, human aging, and age-related diseases. Experimental Gerontology, 39(11–12), 1723–1729. https://doi.org/10.1016/j.exger.2004.04.012.

Laino, C. (n.d.). High-fat diet linked to poor sleep. WebMD. Retrieved January 6, 2023, from https://www.webmd.com/sleep-disorders/news/20080610/high-fat-diet-linked-to-poor-sleep.

Lampiao, F. (2013). New developments of the effect of melatonin on reproduction. World Journal of Obstetrics and Gynecology, 2(2), 8. https://doi.org/10.5317/wjog.v2.i2.8.

Melatonin: What you need to know. (n.d.). NCCIH. Retrieved January 6, 2023, from https://www.nccih.nih.gov/health/melatonin-what-you-need-to-know.

Nesbitt, A. D. (2018). Delayed sleep-wake phase disorder. Journal of Thoracic Disease, 10(S1), S103–S111. https://doi.org/10.21037/jtd.2018.01.11.

O'Connor, A. (2008, June 17). The claim: A spicy meal before bed can disrupt sleep. The New York Times. https://www.nytimes.com/2008/06/17/health/17real.html.

PA-C, S. M. O., MPAS. (2018, August 15). Might coffee be causing your poor sleep? Clinical Advisor. https://www.clinicaladvisor.com/home/the-waiting-room/might-coffee-be-causing-your-poor-sleep/.

Poza, J. J., Pujol, M., Ortega-Albás, J. J., & Romero, O. (2022). Melatonin in sleep disorders. Neurología (English Edition), 37(7), 575–585. https://doi.org/10.1016/j.nrleng.2018.08.004.

Reiter, R. J., Mayo, J. C., Tan, D.-X., Sainz, R. M., Alatorre-Jimenez, M., & Qin, L. (2016). Melatonin as an antioxidant: Under promises but over delivers. Journal of Pineal Research, 61(3), 253–278. https://doi.org/10.1111/jpi.12360.

Saarela, S., & Reiter, R. J. (1994). Function of melatonin in thermoregulatory processes. Life Sciences, 54(5), 295–311. https://doi.org/10.1016/0024-3205(94)00786-1.

Schmidt, M. H., Swang, T. W., Hamilton, I. M., & Best, J. A. (2017). State-dependent metabolic partitioning and energy conservation: A theoretical framework for understanding the function of sleep. PLOS ONE, 12(10), e0185746. https://doi.org/10.1371/journal.pone.0185746.

Scott, A. J., Webb, T. L., & Rowse, G. (2017). Does improving sleep lead to better mental health? A protocol for a meta-analytic review of randomised controlled trials. BMJ Open, 7(9), e016873. https://doi.org/10.1136/bmjopen-2017-016873.

Sleep and body temperature—Are you cool enough? (n.d.). Retrieved January 6, 2023, from https://insomnia-free.com/sleep-and-body-temperature.html.

The best foods to help you sleep. (2017, January 11). Sleep Foundation. https://www.sleepfoundation.org/nutrition/food-and-drink-promote-good-nights-sleep.

U.S. Department of Health and Human Services. (n.d.). Circadian rhythms. National Institute of General Medical Sciences. Retrieved January 6, 2023, from https://www.nigms.nih.gov/education/fact-sheets/Pages/circadian-rhythms.aspx.

Why do we sleep, anyway? | healthy sleep. (n.d.). Retrieved January 6, 2023, from https://healthysleep.med.harvard.edu/healthy/matters/benefits-of-sleep/why-do-we-sleep.

Why do we sleep? (2020, July 20). Healthline. https://www.healthline.com/health/why-do-we-sleep.

Printed in France by Amazon
Brétigny-sur-Orge, FR